FASHION 2.0:

SEASON

OF

CHANGE

A FORECAST OF DIGITAL TRENDS SET
TO DISRUPT THE FASHION INDUSTRY

YULI ZIV

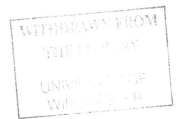

ISBN 978-0615875804

For contact and other info please visit www.YuliZiv.com

Editor: Jim Thomsen

There are many dimensions to the radical shift of this age. People everywhere are talking about it, making predictions or debunking it. Some sense the shift as a cataclysm or end of the world; others as a new beginning; and still others as a time of uncertainty and unpredictability.

We have always experienced change, but rarely with this intensity and speed, and never with this scope and vastness. This change is radical, not incremental. It is a simultaneous change in both outer and inner worlds. The mind is changing its sensitivity, its basic frequency and functioning. Our lifestyle is changing its sense of time, space, relatedness, and relevancy.

~Yogi Bhajan, Ph.D.

Contents

Foreword.

The fashion industry will change more in the next ten years than it has in the last one hundred. The driver of this change will be technology: technology that changes the role of the retailer, technology that changes the capabilities of brands to access their customers, and technology that changes every aspect of consumer behavior. Stepping back to think and speculate how this industry will evolve is a fascinating challenge and this book provides a wonderful cross-sectional view of many impacts from these changes and how they will manifest themselves into all aspects of this industry.

I met Yuli in early 2009 when her Fashion 2.0 Meetup was getting off the ground. As a venture capitalist fascinated by this incredible industry, Fashion 2.0 provided a venue to check the pulse of retail and fashion and to get an early glimpse into some of the companies that hoped to change it. While these meetings were valuable and informative to the many investment theses we were pursuing at First-Mark Capital (we invested in Pinterest, Shopify, and several other companies around this time), the greatest value was the friendship I struck with its fearless leader in whom I found a true kindred spirit regarding the coming revolution in retail. While we did not always agree, the passionate debates helped me coalesce in my mind a vision for this industry that I am pursuing from an investment perspective.

Why a revolution now? Because only now is the true impact of the internet being realized. You are now connected to everyone on the planet who matters to you. Everyone. Any time or all the time. Moreover, you have unlimited computer power at your fingertips to find any answer or perform any analysis you desire. You have unlimited storage to keep a record of anything and everything that is important to you. You have unlimited bandwidth through which you can send any electronic media in any form to anyone. And by the way, on a unit basis, it's almost free. These dynamics are unleashing a wave of creativity of immeasurable magnitude that will impact every aspect of the fashion industry from materials to manufacturing to customer service to marketing to sales to the physical shopping experience and everything in between.

The internet is not just another "door" through which you can sell products to your customer, rather it's the central nervous system through which the entire relationship with the customer is defined. It's not another door: it determines where you put your "doors" and what your doors look like. The store of the future might not be a store, but rather a set of unique experiences that define the "personality" of the brand and enables the brand to touch its customers in a multitude of ways beyond simple display and fulfillment.

For more than a century, the central role of the retailer was to be the gatekeeper between the brand and the customer. The gates are still there, but the internet has torn down the walls that made the gate valuable. Brands can, are and will connect directly with their customers. Retailers who cling to the old gatekeeper model will die but those who embrace this change will thrive not as resellers but as service providers who are invaluable partners who function as service providers existing for only one reason: the success of the brands they support.

Lawrence Lenihan
Managing Director
FirstMark Capital

SEASON

OF

CHANGE

My Life and Change.

One of the reasons this book is so special to me is because of the concept of change, which I've been testing for the majority of my life.

While "life changes" might have a negative connotation for most people who are accustomed to living their lives in a certain way, never leaving their close environment and growing up with the same beliefs for generations, I had no choice but put these beliefs to the test, constantly.

I believe my ability to adapt to change accounts for my professional success. It allows me to navigate my path in this new and constantly changing frontier of digital media.

I spent the first fifteen years of my life absorbing the ideals of Communism, being raised on the principles of equality, hard work and service to country. Terms like *entrepreneurship, building a brand, marketing* and *luxury* simply didn't exist in the Russia of the '70s and '80s. The idea of questioning ideals didn't exist either. Life for the most part was predefined and promised stability—as long as I followed the ideals.

That is, until around 1991, when a period called Perestroika arrived in Russia, and those traditional Communist ideals were shattered. My family and I were forced to escape Russia and take refuge in Israel. There we discovered a whole new world based on completely opposite principles.

The teenaged me couldn't analyze all the aspects of that transformation and come up with a plan to cope with change. But a survival instinct kicked in that allowed me to not only survive, but thrive.

Ironically, I was faced with a whole new set of ideals I had to follow in order to fit into the Israeli society. I served two years in the Israeli Defense Force, only loosely understanding what exactly I was defending. It was certainly a change from life under Communism, but not necessarily for the better.

In 2003, I choose to make another change—to leave Israel and move to New York City, possibly the most fast-paced city on earth. New norms, cultural customs and beliefs made for another major life challenge.

Transforming your life to an entirely new environment once makes you adaptable to change, but doing it twice makes you fearless. It makes you realize that nothing is permanent and everything is subjective to your own perception of reality. You realize that it's not your environment that defines things, but your mind. And things can be constantly redefined, with a simple change of thought.

It is a powerful understanding I've gained, one that's extremely relevant today, as many aspects of our lives shift online. In the online world we have more powers than ever to change, innovate and transform. We have the power to create action among millions of people with a simple message. This is something that no generation before us has been able to do.

Having spent the last six years in the startup world, I saw brilliant ideas being born, being mass-adopted, and then being trashed just a few years later. Companies and brands that were meaningful just a couple of years ago have absolutely no power today. The same rules apply to countries—my homeland, which was one of the most powerful countries in the world in the twentieth century, doesn't have much influence in the new digital world, where physical dominance is less important.

What's important is flexibility of the mind and the ability to innovate in a pace that goes along with the rapid development of new technologies. The transformation it will bring to our lifestyles is so significant that it minimizes all other issues and conflicts in the world.

We aren't talking just about automating the ways products get produced, which the Industrial Revolution brought to us; we are talking about automating our own brain processes and upgrading the human body, processes that haven't changed much since the ancient times. The ability to do so will bring about the era of magical inventions, which some of us will be lucky to not only witness, but conceive.

What does it have to do with fashion, you may ask?

The best part about upgrading our bodies is the preceding process: before we accept the thought of cyber-technology-infused bodies, we will be upgrading the covers of our bodies—our clothes. After all, it is much easier to get behind the idea of Google Glasses than surgically modified eyes connected to the World Wide Web.

We are at the very beginning of an amazing time, where wearable tech will be one of the frontiers of innovation, allowing us to fully integrate technology into our clothes and lifestyles. I can't wait to live the next decade and experience the change. But before we get there, it is important to prepare our minds to the change. Our minds are like a muscle that needs training. They need to be fast and flexible, capable to react quickly and efficiently to any outside changes.

I trained my mind by taking drastic steps, often misunderstood by people around me: moving to new countries, quitting dream jobs, and leaving loved ones. I knew it was necessary for me to evolve, and to flex my mind for the upcoming challenge. In business, I revisit my business model every year or two, examining it against the new reality and making sure it still works. This has been one of the most painful yet most fulfilling exercises I've done—erasing life patterns and building new ones.

To flex your mind, think about simple changes in your life as an exercise for its muscles. Start small by introducing little things that interfere with your daily routine. Continue with bigger spontaneous changes, eventually coming to the place where change is welcome and even creates a sensationally positive reaction in your mind. This is how you know you are ready for this new era.

People and Change.

Let's admit it. Most people are uncomfortable with change. It represents the unknown and could be a major cause of anxiety. Our brains and bodies are naturally built to think in patterns, and even though our lives are constantly in movement, this movement isn't necessarily a change. Most of it is an evolution or morphing of these patterns. Change is breaking the patterns completely and creating new ones. It challenges our reality as we know it.

The change we've experienced in the past decades is something our brains have never experienced before. We've created an artificial intelligence known as a computer, which is based on the patterns of a human brain. Then we created the online space, which is built based on the patterns of our reality. We added a whole new dimension to our existence, which became an integral part of our lives. With all its advantages, this new digital reality has been challenging every area of our lives, introducing changes in every single one of them—the way we communicate, educate, shop, are treated for diseases, and even the way we think.

It has certainly challenged the way we do business.

I believe we are lucky to live in these times of accelerating change. It took humanity centuries to develop the artificial intelligence our computers are using today, but since 1955, when it was officially recognized, the transformation of our lifestyle has been happening at an accelerating—and exciting—pace.

Machines are even allowing us to create our virtual clones, our very own personalities functioning on our behalf in a collective imaginary world—the internet.

We've seen a transformation from manual labor to digitally managed life. We are the first generation who has witnessed such radical change in one lifetime and it is overwhelming.

Some of us are resisting this change and clinging to old values. Some have been consciously ignoring the digital revolution and going back to a simpler, more organic life. But most of us have been trying to adapt. We're being swept away by this digital revolution, realizing there is no way to stop it.

We experience the changes on many different levels—in our private lives, in our relationships with family, friends and co-workers— but especially in our professional lives. Our jobs will never be safe and secure again, because most likely they will be replaced by machines at some point. Most of us, unlike our parents and grandparents, will probably have multiple careers throughout our lifetime, because industries are rapidly redefining themselves and the needs for their workforces are changing.

With this come many challenges.

One of them is the **disorientation and chaos as a result of breaking old hierarchy and rules.** Look at the challenges that big old corporations are facing—from online identity crises to the inability to control their brand messages and manage their employees' online activities. Old rules of marketing, customer service and management simply don't work in the new age.

Companies realize their only value is in people—people who are powering their product (employees) and using it (customers). Suddenly they have to find ways to empower, connect and create transformative experiences for both of these groups to keep them on board with their mission.

In case of the fashion industry, the industry shakeup has started from the media side—the old guard who, for ages, dictated trends, promoted designers and influenced buying decisions was suddenly threatened by millions of individuals with opinions they freely expressed online. There was no one to curate, censor or approve—except the audience. Online readers crave new opinions and new content every day—and they don't care if the content was certified, approved, or even true.

Another very important challenge we are facing is the **free access to information and increasing transparency.** It is hard to control the message in the age when information is free and easily accessible. It is hard to control the sources of information, when everyone is a source.

The viral nature of social media also makes it practically impossible to keep secrets. Almost every moment and every object in this universe is now documented by someone else, and we have to accept that we have little control over the content that people put out there.

Most fashion designers still live in fear of their designs being copied online, or their aura of exclusivity being diminished once they join the online conversation. However, the conversation will be happening, with or without them. Their creations will be knocked off with or without them, because for every great product there is a cheaper alternative. By overprotecting their ideas, they prevent the world from seeing the beauty of their creations and the beauty of the creative process.

Another change-driven challenge is the shift from individualism, to group consciousness that develops online. The growing global awareness teaches us that each individual affects in some way groups of people in different places. This is the era of collective consciousness, in which it is practically impossible to mind your own business, whether you are a country, a company or an individual.

Countries group together to solve problems (European Union), companies become more aware of the environment inside and outside, and individuals become more social. We help strangers fund their dreams via Kickstarter and we create Facebook groups to try to stop governments from making stupid decisions.

We are connected to more groups than ever, via more networks than ever, and these connections will only become deeper as our online and offline activities merge with the help of new technologies.

At the same time, more people are becoming independent and stepping on the entrepreneurial path. People work remotely from different places in the world, or as consultants who are lending their expertise while keeping their personal freedom.

If you have noticed, a lot of people active in social media are of the kind mentioned above. Having a social media presence and persona is a step towards personal freedom, helping us redefine who we are. Many of us build a whole online personality and use it to attract business, educate people or simply entertain.

Fashion Industry and Change.

With this book, my goal is to take a broad look at the transformative changes we are going through, and analyze how these changes are affecting the fashion industry.

How do these digital trends—from social media to wearable tech—affect the way brands are created, businesses run, messages marketed and products are sold? Trying to predict the future might be disturbing for some, and exhilarating for others. But the purpose of this book is not to overwhelm you, but get you prepared for what's to come.

How is the fashion industry adapting to these changes? Why has it been so hesitant to adopt the digital revolution at the beginning? And why is it still resisting in many ways?

Fear is the core reason to why the fashion industry hasn't been swept away by the digital revolution ... yet. In the past few years, it tested the waters and came to accept many of the new rules. However, the biggest changes are still ahead of us, and this is why I wanted to write this book.

I can clearly see this industry changing top to bottom in the next few years, with many roles redefined and even diminished. The reason this change would be so big is because this industry is still dominated by the manual labor on most part.

In this book, I focus on the biggest digital trends we are seeing and how they'll affect the fashion world. I invite you to pause for a moment, between your next spring and fall collections, and recognize those changes. **If you are a fashion designer, executive, marketer, journalist, editor, stylist or blogger, what should be on your mind is not spring or fall season, but the season of change we are going through.**

I realize that it's hard to take time to reflect the changes in the outside world in this fast-paced, obsessed-with-the-next-season industry. The truth is that the technology forecast affecting your production cycle could be more crucial than a color-blocking trend coming back next season. If you can't see where this industry might be in the next ten or twenty years, getting the next fashion trend right won't help you survive. With this book, I invite you to take the journey into the future, imagining together what our careers, shopping experience and clothes are going to look like.

I can hear the skeptics in the corner, asking why they should believe me and my future predictions. Who appointed me to become the Nostradamus of fashion?

No one did. And this is the beauty of the age we live in. We don't need the appointment from above; we can appoint ourselves to become who we want. The rest is taken care of by the tools we created. The new technology allows me to self-publish my thoughts into a book and claim my statements in the biggest bookstore on the planet, called Amazon. There is no editor to decide if my statements are valid or not. People buying my books are the ones validating my place as an author and opinion maker.

After selling thousands of copies of my debut book, *Blogging Your Way to the Front Row*, and getting thank-you letters from all over the world, I'm confident that my self-published opinions matter.

This book is a result of thirteen years of actively working and building businesses in the digital space, trying many different hats from interactive developer to designer. From digital artist experimenting with robotics to creative director working at the top digital agency. From a new immigrant to the CEO of a multi-million-dollar company.

The past five years, I dedicated to the online fashion industry. I've watched this industry evolving from the moment I attended the first New York Fashion Week as an independent fashion blogger, back in 2007. Now I watch it much closer, in my CEO role, running one of the first blogger networks—Style Coalition.

I've worked with Fortune 100 retailers and spoke at countless digital conferences from New York to Moscow. I created the Fashion 2.0 meetup group back in 2008, way before fashion startups became a trend in New York City. It's since grown to 2,500 members and continues building a local community of innovators.

All these experiences allowed me to collect insights on fashion and technology, and use my analytical skills to digest this information into the book that paints the picture of our industry's future. I filled it with ideas for grabs, hoping to inspire entrepreneurs and encourage brands to think like entrepreneurs. You may argue with some statements and question my assumptions. But my goal is not to be right, but provoke thought and foster innovation.

So let's dream together.

CHAPTER ONE:
CONSUMER

One of the main changes we are seeing today is the active role consumers are playing in the life of a brand, from online reviews to crowdsourcing. Today, consumers have the power to make or break a brand. Since fashion industry relies a lot on consumer choices, analyzing the changes in people's behavior affected by the new technology is crucial for understanding the future of this industry.

Meet the New, Empowered Consumer in Charge of Your Business.

Remember when communicating your message to the world meant that you had to get featured in a newspaper, or write a book, or appear on TV?

The common thread among all of these channels is that someone else in the position of power had to approve your message before it was heard. So even though freedom of speech has been advocated for a hundred years, for the first time in the history of our humanity it is a reality. Every individual with an internet connection has the power to communicate their message to millions of people.

There is no need for a magazine editor or a TV producer to approve our messages. Every message has the right to exist in the world. And today, millions of messages are communicated via online channels and consumed by millions of people we've never met. This is a power we've never had before and our generation is the first to take advantage of it.

While many old-school editors, journalists and writers debate the legitimacy of the new order, most of the innovative thinkers are building huge businesses on this new powerful platform. While the media establishment still tries to confuse the public by questioning whether everyone is entitled to an opinion, there is a rise of hugely influential individuals who have no official "credentials" with audiences of millions. While in the past, such people had to be discovered and promoted, these days—if they are persistent and ambitious enough—they can create their own brands and business from scratch. They don't seek anyone's approval; they simply take advantage of the newly available content distribution tools.

In fashion, these newly empowered individuals define and start trends, build online brands and create huge communities of followers. The trend of empowered individuals is spreading through the entire industry and challenging its various parts.

Essentially, consumers are now turned into active participants in the various parts of the industry, from critiquing collections when they just hit the runways to helping in the design and buying process.

We first started seeing the signs of democratization in fashion with independent online media. Bloggers started playing active roles (and in some cases, creating rules) in the three main areas that magazine editors used to rule exclusively—fashion-news coverage, style advice and product recommendation.

News coverage used to be exclusively owned by several trusted publications that would break the news about the latest collections, trends and runway events. While these sources of information still exist, and journalists still have the undeniable power, millions of other sources have been added to them, each blending news reporting with fresh points of view.

Yes, objective reporting still has value when it comes to corporate announcements and business reports, but when it comes to runway news, there is more room for interpretation. Today we see individuals equipped with professional quality cameras or smartphones, contributing to the pool of information. The empowered individuals are now part of the news cycle, whether you accept it or not. They are disrupting the old process with their instant updates, syndicated via multiple viral channels, reaching millions before the "approved" message even has a chance to be processed.

As our connection to technology gets more organic, our devices become more sophisticated, and more skillful individuals rise to the top, we will see better packaged, bite-sized instant news reports competing with the official sources and eventually winning because of two advantages: low barrier to entry, and passion that people can have only when they are fulfilling their own missions.

For years we've been given style advice by a relatively small group of people ruling the industry—editors, magazine writers, stylists and TV hosts. They defined standards and trends, which often lacked diversity or even practicality. They lack that connection to the masses that you can get only by living outside of your industry bubble.

This is where empowered individuals win again. They come in all shapes and colors. They come from diverse backgrounds. They all rise from the bottom, because it's the only way to validate your influence on others—not by being appointed by someone above, but by being voted on by the community who wants to listen. This is a fundamental difference that builds their trust and their power. Empowered individuals rise organically from communities of followers who are thirsty for their expertise, knowledge and experience. They've had the same challenge and managed to overcome it, and now they are sharing it with strangers, and thus becoming closer. Whether it is a plus-size or petite fashion, people trust advice from people who are like them.

Empowered individuals not only give style advice, they move merchandise. For every piece of advice, there are products that go with it. Today these individuals have the opportunity to not only share their advice and products, but monetize this process. People with large online followings are getting premium commissions from brands or networks, essentially becoming virtual salespeople. They essentially help online retailers, who don't have sales people "on the floor" of their e-commerce destinations.

All an e-commerce brand needs these days is an endorsement of an empowered individual to move the product off their virtual shelves. Again, while media is still arguing the ethical side of affiliate sales, individual bloggers have been making thousands of dollars through product recommendations within their editorial content. And now, even magazines are jumping on the trend.

This is why we will also see more technology solutions that will allow individuals to monetize their influence. As online retail continues to grow, the key to success will lie in seamless process, allowing the influencers to earn revenue from multiple platforms without much effort.

This is where some of the biggest opportunities for technology exist: we have many tools empowering individuals, but fewer ways to monetize their influence. Technology that will allow the real and seamless rewarding of the influential individuals will be extremely powerful.

How the Self-Publishing Revolution is Challenging Media Corporations.

Empowered individuals wouldn't have been so influential if they didn't have the tools that allow them to express themselves and build their audiences.

The online publishing revolution started in 1999, with two companies that gave birth to the blogging trend: LiveJournal, started in April 1999 by programmer Brad Fitzpatrick as a way of keeping his high school friends updated on his activities; and Blogger, launched by Pyra Labs in August 1999. As one of the earliest dedicated blog-publishing tools, Blogger is credited for helping popularize the format, which later disrupted many industries outside the publishing world.

Today with publishing options ranging from WordPress and Tumblr to Pinterest, Instagram, Vine, Twitter and Amazon, publishing anything from quick thoughts to magazines and novels couldn't be easier. However what made online publishing really powerful is the rise of social media, which allowed individuals to build large-scale audiences of fans to consume their content.

Suddenly, individuals are empowered not only with self-expression tools that turned them into broadcasting media sources,

but thanks to social networks, they are also equipped with distribution channels. They are becoming media empires on their own right. In the age of low barrier to entry into online publishing, they can build multi-million dollar businesses, and do it without investing a penny just by using the free tools available online.

Back in 2010, when I decided to self-publish my first book, I did not realize how accessible it was. I invested nothing but my own time in the book, and a few months later the final product was available for anyone in the world to buy via the world's largest books distributor — Amazon. Five years ago, I wouldn't have believed you if you told me this would be possible.

These new turnkey technologies don't just empower individuals; they give them superpowers to be an all-in-one publishing company—artist, author, editor, publisher and distributor. Today, any talented individual has all the tools to compete with an established publisher, and many do so successfully. In doing so, they challenge the old ways of thinking and doing business.

We are seeing more journalists and editors quitting their corporate jobs to build their own authority and brand online. This trend will only continue to grow, breaking up the old hierarchies even more and allowing individuals to group together into companies and publications, unlike in the past when a corporation would group together individuals.

This is the principle upon which I built my company, Style Coalition. Often called the Condé Nast of the new generation, we grouped several independent online publishers with distinct voices that represent large and diverse audiences. Style Coalition's mission is to monetize the content and advertising space, and save publishers the burden of building a sales and advertising operations team. Each site can focus on being the best in its category—an influential, inspiring publication—and share the business resources with other similar publications, just like big publishing companies do. Instead of the top-down approach cultivated for years by corporations, we have built the company on the principals of empowered individuals who we help grow.

These days more companies than ever adopt this approach. Kickstarter became the ultimate channel to fundraise for ideas—in fashion, many aspiring designers are using it to fund their first collections. CreateSpace and Amazon are empowering individuals to publish books, and SkillShare empowers everyone to become a teacher and share their unique knowledge.

The examples are endless and touch most aspects of our lives. **Today we have all the tools needed to pursue our dreams. The barriers to entry will continue to lower and coming up with excuses for not pursuing your ideas will be harder and harder.**

Why Consumers Know Better
and How to Utilize Their Knowledge.

Consumer influence on brands doesn't stop at simply expressing opinions on products; it is becoming an integral part of product design and functionality.

Since the Industrial Revolution and the establishment of mass production, brands got used to the idea of coming up with a new product idea, manufacturing it, then trying to market and sell to potential customers. Until recently, fashion retailers relied on the expertise of merchants and buyers to identify designs with the most commercial potential.

Social media is challenging this concept. By having direct connection to consumers, brands can involve them in the product decisions at the very early stage. Some even crowd-source ideas, by asking brand fans for advice on shape, color, cut and more.

It can be argued that in fashion, consumers never know what they actually want or need until they see and like it. That is true to some extent, especially when it comes to new trends introduced by designers. High fashion will always exist as a form of art and will continue to inspire us just like a beautiful painting does.

However, most people in their everyday life tend to stick to the same types of fashion products. People will always buy pants, because our body has two legs. People will always buy hats because we need to protect our head and our heads have a round shape. So the basic product types will stay the same; however, they could be greatly optimized with the help of consumers.

By involving consumers in the design process, brands may discover issues that never occurred to them, simply because people have a different body shape or live in a different climate. By inviting consumers to participate in the creative process, brands are turning clothes-wearers into loyal fans, personally involved in the final result.

Crowdsourcing is part of the same democratization trend we are seeing in all parts of the industry. Instead of the top-down approach of "We will tell you what to wear next spring," the conversation is changing to "Tell us what you would prefer to wear next spring." We can see the beginning of the change when fashion brands use early runway photos and the number of "likes" on each as an indication of purchase interest, and change their production quantities accordingly.

Now imagine if you could save the effort of creating samples and sending them down an expensive runway early in the design process—and instead showcase only the winning products, which got the most votes from a brand's loyal fans? The thought may look irrational to avid fashion fans, who are attached to the idea of surprise and mystery when it comes to the design process.

But most fashion brands are first and most are businesses that need to care about their spending and profit margins. This is where the idea of consumer participation may save money. Imagine producing only items that consumers want, and not wasting the effort on something people not only never wanted but will never buy.

In the technology startup industry, this concept is known as MVP—a Minimal Viable Product needed to prove the use and purchase intent. In the early internet days, engineers would work on a fully functioning product, perfecting it for years before release, only to find out that their assumptions were off about who would want it.

Today we see startup companies launch with just a single web page. They gauge user interest and continue developing their fully functioning products while implementing the feedback. This approach saves not only time and money, but allows useful, desirable brands to develop.

Similarly, a designer or a brand may work passionately on a new piece of clothing only to find out that no one wants to wear it, and their exquisite creation ends up in an outlet store, to be sold at a fraction of its actual cost. We criticize fast-fashion retailers for lowering production standards and pricing on apparel, while on average, a small percentage of designer merchandize is sold at its full price.

People who criticize the fast-fashion concept often ignore the important role of a consumer, driving these businesses with their demand. Fast-fashion companies like Zara are using customer feedback to build more efficiency. Sales representatives in store locations are used to gain consumer feedback and report back so the retailer can adjust anything from colors and shapes, as well as send more quantities to the locations in the world where certain products are more popular.

Of course they are able to respond to the demand quickly because of the fast way their items are produced. Most fashion brands tend to look down at this strategy of constantly producing garments instead of releasing four to six seasonal collections, like most brands do.

Those who analyze this idea through the lenses of constant change and the pace we live in might think that Zara is brilliant and ahead of times in its approach. Instead of relying on the old rules of the retail industry, Zara created its own rules. It responded to change by fully embracing change, realizing its consumer lives not in the fall or spring, but in the season of change. It builds its business by catering to that change. Perhaps that's the reason the company is now valued at $8 billion?

Technology and social media brings us closer to our audience and consumers, and that allows brands to continue adjusting their products and become more useful and efficient. This new approach completely changes the way brands used to think about their products, and therefore is difficult for most to accept. I truly believe that brands that come down off their pedestals, and be open and inclusive with their consumers, will see a huge return.

We are seeing how this pays off now on a small scale, with brands becoming more approachable and communicating with fans on Twitter and Facebook. Right now, however, there is still a culture of behind-the-scenes and insider-only access surrounding the fashion industry. Most fashion brands still believe in the idea of mystique as the driver of consumer interest. But that veil will be eventually unveiled, challenged by the law of motion.

Fashion companies can choose to stay at the station, but that doesn't mean the entire world will stay there too. The pace of change has been exponentially increasing, soon reaching the Singularity point, which I'll be touching upon in the next chapters. My best advice to brands that question the new order is to develop flexibility and courage, or the viability of their businesses will be challenged from every direction.

How We Lost Our Privacy, aka the Best Thing Happened to Innovation.

The openness with which people communicate online is one of the reasons consumers are becoming so powerful. They don't comprise just a silent mass of people with credit cards who either buy or don't buy a product; they are opinionated individuals who have the tools to express their opinions and they control the distribution channels to make these opinions influential.

They aren't hiding behind anonymous nicknames, as they did in the early internet days. They are not only proud of their opinions; they want these opinions to be attached to their names. By forming their original opinions online, they are attracting followings and building their influence. This influence is a valuable asset which today can be rewarded and even monetized. Being rewarded usually outweighs the privacy concerns or shyness that stopped some in the early days.

Trust is the highest currency in the virtual world, and having a trusting audience listening to your opinions has a tremendous value, no matter what you do. If you are expressing opinions on news and events and have a trusting audience, you can monetize your opinions via advertising.

Likewise, if you are expressing opinions about products and thus influencing purchasing decisions, your opinions have tremendous value to these brands.

To gain the audience trust, you have to be open. You have to show your human side, whether it's positive or negative. It is the only way people can relate. We see more people doing just that online— exposing anything from their divorces to their controversial opinions, because it's impossible to create a following by trying to please every- one. People are attracted to unique points of view.

Some people choose to expose themselves, and some are being exposed without their will. Transparency is another blessing and a curse of the age of openness we live in. Truth comes out easier and faster than ever, because our lives are documented in so many ways, whether we want it or not. Celebrities are being documented by the paparazzi and the rest of us are being documented by our smartphone-equipped friends.

The only way to hide from this is to live on a distant island with- out an online connection. Otherwise you will have to accept the fact that your privacy will be exposed. You can fight it by controlling your privacy settings on Facebook or other social platforms you use, but **essentially the web is one big public billboard of our activities,** and everything and anything is prone to be exposed at some point.

You can argue that, but the process has already begun and is now progressing. Almost every online activity is tracked by cookies, internet providers, GPS, or our own followers. It is impossible to hide in the digital age.

Essentially, we are moving towards a complete loss of privacy, and the new generation is a great example to that process. It's a transformation of our collective mind that is already affecting society on a larger level, and certain groups like celebrities are also affected on a personal level. We see more of their secrets revealed and more private stories becoming major news. **When the world is connected and tracked by technology, keeping secrets becomes challenging.**

At the same time, people consume more "shocking" private information—and share their own with others. The act of public exposure loses its novelty and becomes just another piece of information we consume daily. Transparency becomes an integral layer of our lives. It is also slowly becoming an essential part of our businesses.

Essentially, innovation is winning over our fear of privacy. The benefits will slowly outweigh the concerns.

What does it mean for brands? A huge opportunity to connect with their consumers on a deeper level. By knowing private details about their customers' lives and personalities, brands can tailor customized products or offerings for them. And that will lead to better customer experiences.

For a long time, brands were seeing the consumer as a mass of people, having a stereotypical character in mind. Often fashion designers would describe that person in terms such as "an urban girl in her early twenties, she is on the go, with a busy schedule and rich social life who needs a quick solution for day-to-night wardrobe." These stock descriptions become laughable in the age of social media, when designers have the opportunity to connect with that "girl" on her social media channels and discover that each consumer has a different personality and different needs. Today we can gather the data to know exactly who these people are, from their age and marital status to their dress size and favorite movies.

Most brands are still in the stage of simply aggregating this data without putting much of it to use—for example, personalization of their offers. There aren't many plug-and-play technologies that can do that automatically ... yet. But in the next couple of years, we will see more tools allowing brands to not only track but build deeper relationships with the consumers.

Facebook has revolutionized social media by combining these two functions: the ability to track and receive data, and the ability to build deeper personal connections. However it could not crack the code on the last piece of that cycle—selling a product. After opening their Facebook stores a couple of years ago, they were abandoned not long after by most brands.

While consumers are used to the idea of having relationships with brands on their social media platforms, the Facebook stores didn't offer anything different from the traditional e-commerce channels. They didn't combine the personal data with offerings that provided a better customer experience. And this is something brands will have to fix in the next few years as technology gets more sophisticated.

In the future, all of us won't be seeing the same homepage on Saks.com. We each will see our own Saks.com, customized to our style, our taste and our wallet. Think about the efficiency of showing customers only the colors they love, in the sizes that fit them and the styles that reflect their everyday life.

In fact, I believe if we built the web today from scratch, this would be the natural experience we would think about creating. Yes, somehow our online retail got stuck in the static HTML days, realizing only a fraction of its potential. In online retail, we still lack the social layer, along with dynamic pricing and personalization. All are huge opportunities for technology companies.

Consumers are willing to share data in order to get a personalized experience; we are past the point of hesitation. According to a recent study in the U.K., 75 percent of consumers who have an existing relationship with a company are happy to share their information with it, while 62 percent would share their information with a company selling products or services they need.

This might be the biggest and most underestimated opportunity for brands today. Thanks to the lifted veil of personal privacy, they have direct access to their core fans. That gives them an opportunity to research them and understand them better, to build more meaningful relationships and offer a much better experience.

CHAPTER TWO:
BRAND

This new reality in which consumers have more power than ever, in which social media is one of the major communication channels and transparency is one of the most valued qualities, presents many challenges to brands. They are tasked with opening up, with reinventing business practices, and with changing the way they market their products. It is hard to be a brand in an age when people skip commercials; however, it is easier than ever to build real relationships with consumers. The only question is, are brands ready to commit to these relationships?

Brands are Getting a Personality.

How does a brand participate in this new online reality built on personal relationships, direct communication and trust? All these terms refer to connections between people, not people and logos. Today it is getting harder for brands to hide behind logos, mission statements and communication guidelines. The only way to participate in the online conversation effectively is by having a personality.

How does a brand with thousands of workers find its personality? Some are lucky to be founded by visionaries, who are closely associated with the brand and are their natural spokespeople. Some hire a celebrity to speak on their behalf. Some empower their employees to become brand spokespeople in social media. **All these strategies point to the rising trend of personification.**

If you look at the most successful brand examples in social media, they all possess human qualities, even if their personality is fictional or split among multiple people representing the brand. Brands like Tory Burch, Diane Von Furstenberg and Marc Jacobs were lucky to have designers behind them who felt comfortable sharing their lives and thoughts on social media. Millions of fans love these brands and personalities enough to tune in daily and follow their updates, which include anything from vacation with the kids to a day at their studio.

DKNY, whose founder Donna Karan does not personally use social media, was one of the first to dive into it by creating a character that is a perfect combination of a fashion industry insider and every girl's best friend. She is a typical New Yorker who can never catch a cab, is obsessed with *Gossip Girl*, and calls 4 p.m. a "candy hour." Naturally, the character creates so many points for identification that the followers feel a strong connection to the brand via its virtual personality.

This perfectly illustrates one of the main brand strategies for online communications in the era of personification: **solidarity**. Being able to make people relate to your brand's character in a very personal way, having common traits and sharing similar challenges creates a powerful bond that lifts the brand to the status of a person, not just a logo. People feel like they are communicating with a real person and forget that it is a commercial brand with a line of products behind it.

Today it is not enough to just have product attached to your brand name. You have to have a set of personal values attached to it as well. In the age of social media, people's perception of your brand is based not only on the quality of your products and creativity of your collection, it is based on the personality your brand projects—via its founders, executives, employees, spokespeople and all people involved with the brand.

In order to stay in the game brands must use their personality to earn the love of consumers. In social media, love is expressed in multiple ways. On Twitter, love is measured by the number of followers and re-tweets. On Facebook, it's by the number of page fans. On Pinterest, it's by the number of pins with the brand name. No one has yet combined these metrics and come up with the formula to measure this form of brand affection. But everyone now understands the importance of it.

No expensive TV commercial or beautiful magazine ad could give a chance to consumers to express their love for brands and build relationship. The only way to do so is via social media. Unlike advertising, social conversations are a two-way street and have the potential to lead to close personal relationships. In our day and age, these relationships with the consumer are the hottest brand commodity. Whether they need to buy or earn consumers love, this is something brands can't afford to ignore.

"Are You Talking to Me?" or
The End of Top-down Marketing.

How does a brand who has a personality market its products? Certainly not via pre-packaged promotional messages. These include TV commercials that interrupt our favorite shows for thirty seconds. It also includes intrusive banner ads covering the content we are trying to consume online.

Of course, there are still entertaining commercials out there. The best of them are celebrated during the Super Bowl, but let's admit it — most of them are just desperate screams for customers' attention.

The advertising industry today is in most part relying on the idea of capturing the consumer in a moment of weakness and ambushing them with a message about a product they didn't know they needed. Hours of research go into finding out when and where that weakest moment happens — is it when the person is watching TV after a long day at the office, or while they are reading content online? Once the weakest moment is identified, the person gets forced to pay attention to the marketing message — on TV in the most aggressive way by interrupting a favorite show, or online by distracting with flashy banners.

It's a known fact that it takes a person seven times to be exposed to the message in order to remember it. You might as well sedate them and program your marketing message into their brain.

The advertising tactics worked for a few decades now, but as technology innovation is progressing, people get inventive about tuning out—from DVR devices to banner blockers, they've been putting up a good fight for a few years now. You can force people to do something they never wanted only for so long. Eventually they rebel. And marketers will have to find other, more creative ways to get their attention.

Social media gave a chance for brands and marketers to stop screaming and interrupting their customers—and instead, interact and engage. Brands could become part of the conversation and promote their products in the relevant parts of this conversation, on Facebook, Twitter, Instagram, Pinterest and many other platforms.

Content marketing or native advertising is another channel brands have been adopting. It is also something I've been involved in for the past few years, helping brands to connect to relevant influencers and share brand stories via these influential voices. Interestingly enough, in the four-year history of Style Coalition, none of our campaigns ever got a negative response from readers or was called intrusive advertising. Often we witness the opposite—readers thanking bloggers for helping them find good products via sponsored stories they shared on the blog.

Social media forced the brands to adapt to this new environment, in which they became part of the conversation, but were not the only participants. Consumers could finally talk back.

If marketers can overcome the risk factor that goes into opening up, they will be able to see the advantages of finally knowing what people really think about their brand and product. Social media is a blessing that's going to save all of us from being aggressively attacked by advertising.

I can see how some of you would disagree—after all, our Facebook pages are already flooded by marketers. However, I believe what we are witnessing now is a period of transformation, a learning curve in which people are testing the boundaries. You can see how quickly aggressive brands get outed on Facebook in the most negative ways. The more #socialmediafails we witness, the more these brands will learn and eventually come up with a way to communicate that provides value to others.

As you know, great businesses and great products don't need aggressive advertising—yes, they might need marketing in forms of product-seeding and education, but they never try to put their customer in a chair and yell their message seven times until the person gets it.

My hope with this book is to turn my readers into the second group—marketers and business people who look at their audience as a collection of unique individuals, not a "target group." Because of the marketing philosophies we've been following for years, we lost the ability to communicate on an individual level. We glamorized the concept of going after masses, instead of first trying to change the life of a single individual.

In fashion, designers are trying to compete with each other over who can reach more masses, instead of trying to make the lives of individuals more colorful, beautiful, and comfortable. If they spent the same amount of resources they spend today on top-down advertising, thinking of how they could create a better value for their customer and their brands would be naturally more admired.

Heritage is Marketers' Best Lie,
or Why Luxury Brands are in Trouble.

When it comes to century-old luxury brands like Louis Vuitton, Hermes and Cartier, *heritage* is a common term used in every list of brand values and every brand mission written by their marketers. "You can't compete with one hundred years of brand heritage," they say.

It is true that history is an important part of every brand, especially if you can make it relevant for today's consumer. However, it would be much harder to make the new generation of consumers born in the digital age excited about a hundred years of heritage and craftsmanship. What they will care about is how cool a product is among their peers, how innovative it is, and how it solves their daily style challenges.

We are seeing brands born online and manage to build millions of customers and millions of dollars in revenues within just a year or two. The new generation of online brands like Gilt, Fab, FarFetch and Net-A-Porter don't have a heritage attached to their names—and they are surpassing the growth of any traditional retailer with a long list of loyal customers.

How do you explain this phenomenon? **Innovation is slowly replacing heritage as the new attribute of luxury.** Ironically enough, it represents the opposite idea of the heritage—an idea of the future, not the past. Jumping a few years ahead, hiding behind heritage won't work when competitive brands will start making digitally wired clothing and use dirt-resistant fabrics. The only reason the hundred years of heritage might matter is if the history was used to innovate the product.

In the digital age, heritage doesn't have as much power, and it certainly doesn't make a brand bulletproof. In fact, it somewhat puts it in a disadvantageous position.

Unlike young brands that can be flexible and easily adapt to change, luxury brands—despite a couple of exceptions—have been holding to their old values, since that's been written on their flag for generations. It is harder for them to admit that things are changing when their entire brand is based on history, heritage and old values.

Another challenge to sustain in this new reality is the craftsmanship—the manual labor that goes into the creations of most luxury labels. They pride themselves in handmade work done by artisans. It's one of the reasons these products are so expensive.

The manual labor is again the exact opposite of the "age of the machines" we are entering. As 3-D printers are becoming a commodity and the sign of the next industrial revolution, the value of manual labor will not only diminish, it will be perceived as a sign of inefficiency.

Why would you employ thirty artisans in South of France who together make three thousand stitches a day, if an average fashion printer of the future would probably be able to make three million stitches per day less than a decade from now?

Luxury brands need to find a new story to tell, before heritage will turn into a disadvantage. They need to focus their significant resources on innovation and lead the industry, instead of holding to the past.

We still see major luxury brands like Chanel resisting e-commerce. According to their leaders, "it can't replicate the personal in-store experience." The truth is they chose not to invest resources in replication of that experience with technology. Ask every Twitter addict if their experience online is personal enough, and most of them will admit it's very real.

If luxury brands followed the same standards and spent as much resources on their website architecture as they use on their over-the-top retail stores, we would be seeing e-commerce masterpieces with engaging experiences, precise fits and personalized offerings.

Of course it's easier to blame the digital world for its two-dimensionalism than it is to try to pioneer the medium. Unfortunately, this is also the most certain way to die in the era we are entering.

The next few years will be the real test for the luxury brands, as their flexibility and the ability to adopt to change will be widely tested.

The most inventive will survive.

Trademarks are Being Killed by Innovation.

The main reason many of the fashion brands and designers were hesitant about social media at first? Fear of revealing too much information and feeding the copycats.

While giving fans a sneak peek into a collection is a great tool to create anticipation and emotional connection, it is also a great inspirational tool for copycats. Whether it's a manufacturer in China knocking off a collection or a competing fast-fashion chain, the damage will be done.

Intellectual property has never been harder to protect than in the information age. Having millions of people accessing your information can have many advantages, but can also create a playground for stolen ideas. Business models get replicated and companies, not to mention individual products, get knocked off.

We are seeing many of the major brands spending months in courtrooms, fighting for their ideas. The trademark registry and patent office are still doing brisk business. Meanwhile, it becomes easier and easier to research and get ideas online. Think about the major force of innovation that is behind new product releases, versus the slow, multi-year process of patents and trademarks and the costly fights in courts that often last years.

If you were a fashion designer or a brand, where would you rather focus your energy and resources? In courts and patent offices, or in your studio coming up with products so amazing that no one can replicate them?

If a brand's product is so easy to replicate, perhaps something unique is missing. Perhaps it is lacking that secret sauce that makes their product unmatched. Yes, dresses are easier to replicate than iPhones, but maybe that's a sign that the dress should be much more "smart" as a product? Think about all the unique techniques and inventions that could make a dress impossible to copy.

The idea of accessible, inexpensive production created a low barrier to entry into the fashion world. Being a draping expert just doesn't cut it anymore. Fashion products need a serious upgrade in order to be different and non-replicable. They require a complete upgrade, turning them from disposable items into long-lasting, smart products that can function for years, just like our gadgets do.

From this perspective, wasting time on patenting the color of a shoe sole is less productive than inventing a color-changing sole. However, painting a sole in red is much easier than installing a digital layer that changes the sole to any color, via remote control. It's much easier, and that's part of a larger problem.

This industry is so caught up in its own bubble, its own fast-paced production cycle, that no one has time to stop and think. Look at the world around and see how it's changed in the past decade. And how little our clothes did.

In fact, we've been mainly recycling trends from the '60s, '70s, '80s and '90s, merely by changing color schemes. Our fabrics still wrinkle and stain and get ruined after just a few laundry cycles. All of this happens in the same world in which people explore space and invent artificial intelligence.

So why does an everyday object used by the entire human race see so little innovation?

Things are about to change and the new pace of innovation will eventually catch up with the fashion industry. Things will be changing so fast and get outdated so fast that there will be no value in patents, and the idea of intellectual property will be replaced by a collective intelligence.

The question that people will be asking themselves won't be "How can I protect my knowledge in order to create the most value for myself?" but "How can I effectively share my knowledge in order to contribute to the collective intelligence and create more value for myself and others?"

This may sound idealistic now, but as our collective consciousness develops, people will feel less need to exercise their own egos and will find that they gain more by acting as a collective with similar goals.

Social media has a huge role in this group-consciousness development. It is in the core of everything from viral videos to trending hashtags. Notice how every time someone—a brand, a celebrity or one of your friends—tries to exercise their own ego in social media, they get a backlash. However, it's never been easier to rally people for any cause, be it commercial or nonprofit.

Recognizing the group consciousness and tuning into it will make it easier to navigate the space, whether you are a brand with a million followers or a follower of million brands.

From Factories to APIs.

The same collective consciousness that's driving the rise of social media and the openness that comes with it will cause brands to re-examine their business values based on competitiveness and trade secrets. To innovate, brands need more efficiency. Efficiency is hard to optimize on a brand level. The change needs to come from the industry as a whole. There is a need for new platforms that provide shared resources that unite everyone in the industry.

The same way Facebook Connect allows any website to easily create user accounts and access user data without developing much on their own, the fashion industry could use a similar approach to design and production. Basic patterns, fabrics, sourcing and production could be accessible via a centralized platform. But it doesn't yet exist.

This is a major barrier to entry in this industry, and an innovation-stopper. After all, it's hard to come up with revolutionary products when the production of a single garment requires so much research, resources, and trial and error. Sharing these basic resources and making them easily accessible to any designer or brand may introduce much-needed efficiency and allow them to focus on pushing limits.

Sharing something as proprietary as design patterns requires brands to open their mind. It also requires them to realize that their real value is not in dress patterns or connections to factories in China;

their value is in creativity of their minds, in signature products that make people feel good, and in a brand image that people want to support.

Just like with the Facebook Connect release, people questioned the business decision of sharing user information with other businesses. Opening up its database, however, and allowing other companies to build businesses on top of their robust platform-accelerated innovation rooted Facebook much more deeply as one of the most powerful companies in the world.

Since then the concept of API (Application Programming Interface) has been adopted by many web companies, which create libraries of data and provide access to it. Some are free and some cost thousands of dollars. But the API approach became a standard in web development, and most web products we use today rely on external APIs in some way.

Sharing data is a new concept for fashion brands, one that hasn't been explored yet. However, as with many digital trends, they usually start among tech communities and eventually get adopted by other industries. I believe the concept of API will be one step toward the revolutionizing of fashion industry.

CHAPTER THREE: RETAIL

Digital innovation not only changed the way brands and consumers interact, but created a set of different shopping habits that now affect online and offline retail. Consumers have more options than ever for researching items and comparing prices. They also have access to the largest collection of products they ever wished for, no matter where in the world they are. They are able to shop for items they love regardless of brand, season or location. The limitless world of online shopping creates new rules affecting the entire food chain — from forecasting and trends to pricing and production.

Retail Turns Interactive.

Fashion brands will go through major transformation in the next decade. So the retail environment will have to change as well. While the department stores of the future will be more like an Apple Store and less like a bazaar overloaded with endless merchandise, there is still a long way to go. The concept of Less Is More was never the fashion industry's favorite. So much must change before we can shop in the store of the future: a gallery-like environment selling an all-in-one digital dress, with several customization options to allow consumers to choose features and compatibility with other wearable devices.

However the beginning of technology innovation is already underway in retail. Retail is turning interactive, thanks to consumers equipped with smartphones and other mobile devices. Retailers are finally realizing the power of data they can gather with the help of technology, which will allow them to optimize the experience as well as entertain the consumer.

Virtual fitting rooms have been tested in several retail locations, removing the need for physical fitting rooms and allowing the shoppers to see the merchandise in a mirrored screen. In the fall of 2012, Microsoft showcased its virtual fitting room technology, based on Kinect and developed by FaceCake in Bloomingdales stores in New

York City. While the concept was more of a temporary pop-up store, it is close to becoming affordable reality.

Other interactive technologies, like the one developed by New York-based Perch, are looking to add interactive layers to displayed products. When a customer touches a bag on display, for example, a projected layer of information pops up, mimicking the same experience of "more info" that we are so used to seeing while shopping online.

San Francisco-based ShopFlick is focusing on mobile retail rewards, integrating them seamlessly into the store-browsing experience. Consumers get alerted on special offers while browsing store merchandise. It's the perfect time to catch their attention.

These technologies make the interactive layer seamless, presenting the relevant shopping information either through in-store devices or consumer-handled mobile phones.

This concept of constant connection to a customer through devices introduces a great opportunity to create unique custom in-store experiences. The much-buzzed-about Gamification is finally coming to physical retail, and we will be seeing more game-like experiments that engage consumers in stores and online. Retailers will be adapting strategies from online game developers to improve the "stickiness" of their in-store customers, by creating engaging, rewarding experiences.

One of the main benefits of this new layer of interaction is the multiple data points collected about the customer and their shopping experience. They allow the retailers to study their behavior and optimize the offering based on that.

New York City-based Placemeter collects retail location data from sensor-powered devices installed in stores. Their technology provides detailed reports with insights on foot traffic by store areas and average time spent by customers. Retailers are then able to analyze the data and improve shoppers experience accordingly.

While many would say some of these technologies have a scary "Big Brother" character to them, the increasing openness of people to the sharing of information gives them a real chance to succeed.

Modern shoppers are used to the idea of information-sharing online; now it's only a matter of time to get them used to the same idea offline. Rewards and incentives already driving retail make it a much easier task.

What Could Retailers Learn From Stock Brokers?

One of the first areas in retail affected by the online web was pricing. It's cheaper than ever to manufacture clothing and the options are wider than we've ever had, which drove down the costs of a simple dress at a mass retailer to as low as $30. Of course, this was made possible because of the Industrial Revolution and the new technological inventions that both improve the production process and the materials used for clothing and footwear. But the web and e-commerce have challenged the prices in many ways as well.

It is easier than ever to make a price comparison for the same product, or compare similar items with different price points. Only a few years ago, the only option for a customer looking for a black T-shirt was going to the local mall, checking out a few stores and buying the best possible product out of these few options. These days, thanks to shopping search engines, the possibilities are endless (to be precise, my online search for a black T-shirt returned 694,091 results, ranging from $3.99 from Hanes to $236 at Gucci). This means the customer has a better chance to find a lower-priced product.

In addition, there is a slew of websites dedicated to finding discounted merchandise. From fashion blogs recommending "The Look for Less" to coupon sites promoting discounts, the web is a paradise for a bargain shopper.

The new generation of online retailers even uses innovative business models focusing on bargains. From flash sale sites like Gilt, ideeli and Rue La La that make shopping a competitive sport, to rental services like Rent the Runway—shopping for new clothes in local stores is not the only option for today's consumer.

Product pricing, in the history of retail industry, has always been inconsistent, and sometimes irrational. How can technology change it? Imagine a stock market-like pricing model, using real-time data to dynamically define pricing.

Consumers are already participating in many aspects of the products—from funding (crowdfunding) to design (crowdsourcing) and marketing (social media). Consumers may eventually decide how much they are willing to pay.

Online auctions aren't new to the web. But they mainly operate the secondhand market, with eBay being the biggest and greatest example of all. On the other end, we are seeing sites like Moda Operandi offering pre-orders of limited quantities of yet-to-be-made merchandise. Marrying the two business models could create an open market for fashion goods, in which items are sold for what they are worth, instead of being overpriced by designers and later sold by retailers at a heavy discount. This inefficient process, in which both parties often lose money, could be solved by technology and real-time bidding.

What dynamic pricing will do is balance the market and prevent the customer from getting the product at the wrong value, which happens often today. There is a race to get products at a lower value, and people brag about getting high-end designer goods at a fraction of a price. Discount retailers are striving. Designers are cornered and thus take profit cuts in a world in which customers find their products in a variety of price points.

Dynamic pricing will allow unity of price points across the web and put a real value on the product. **That product value may be based on production cost, on a brand's profit margin, on quality, on quantities created and on customer demand.**

Right now, the customer is left in the dark about product quality—a $30 dress at Forever 21 is different from a heavily discounted designer dress sold for $30 at Century 21. They are also left in the dark about production quantity, which may affect the price they are willing to pay. In fashion, high value is placed on one-of-a-kind or limited-edition items, so many people will pay higher prices if they knew that the chance of seeing someone else on the street wearing the same things is rare.

Imagine the fashion labels operating in a stock market-type environment, in which the price for Donna Karan gowns may soar after being seen on the red carpet at the Oscars ceremony. Or Marc Jacobs's social media activity and huge following may create a higher demand for a certain item, causing its price to rise.

The same with designers whose collections are just not in demand this season—instead of waiting for the season's end to discount the merchandise or move the inventory to discount retailers, dynamic pricing can measure demand in real time and suggest new valuation. Technology will make this process as efficient as bidding on online advertising placements with Google Adsense. One dashboard could allow you to estimate brand value and adjust pricing. This may take years to introduce to market, and to digitize all of our clothes, but the process is inevitable as we move toward greater efficiency in our life and digitization of all objects. With the high cost of designer goods, there is no reason that brands won't invest in technology—from price adjustment and real-time analytics—that allows them more control over their product, and that eventually will increase their margins.

Why Would You Search
if You Could Simply Discover?

The psychological drivers behind shopping activity have fascinated me for several years now. I've been helping brands connect to their online audiences via the group of influential bloggers my company, Style Coalition, represents. I watched the growth of bloggers' influence on readers' purchasing decisions. And now, blogs now influence 31 percent of overall purchases.

I also watched the way my own shopping habits changed through the years. I've slowly come to the place where 80 percent of my purchases are done online. The idea of offline retail with crowds, lines, busy salespeople, missing sizes and countless clothing racks could never be less appealing. Tools like ShopStyle allow shoppers to find exactly what they want, in just a few clicks. However the biggest appeal of fashion is offering things we didn't know even existed. So how do we discover new products in the online age?

Over the past few years, there has been an underlying shift in the roles we play when it comes to technology. We are moving away from user-initiated (search) to auto-serving (suggestions) technologies, and it's about to change the way we communicate, shop and collaborate. As our online profiles become more sophisticated and mobile tools allow real-time interaction, instead of actively searching for things we will be presented with them, as we live our lives.

We will slowly build trust and allow more technologies to shape our discovery and decision processes. As these technologies become more integral to our lives, search as an activity will become less relevant.

Most of the applications and platforms we use these days require our initiation and action. In order to achieve anything, we have to acknowledge the need, make a decision, and then follow through.

Example: You need a new swimsuit for the summer and you decide to find one that best matches your search criteria: color, style, size, etc. You use Google, ShopStyle, TheFind, or any other smart shopping engine. This simple task requires a bit of thought and effort on your part.

What if you could skip this process and let technology offer you the perfect swimsuit once the summer season arrives, without asking you to take any action? Most of our purchases could be easily predicted as they rely on seasons, our user profile or actions we take.

Location-based apps like Foursquare are halfway there. To enjoy the rewards and badges of this location-based game, users are still required to manually "check in" at various places via GPS-enabled phones. However Foursquare is talking about automating in the future. Once Foursquare overcomes the user-initiation block, it will be able to offer you places on the go, according to your preferences. Are you on the corner of 34th Street and Sixth Avenue in New York City? There is a flagship Victoria's Secret store, and according to your last check-ins, you are a fan of the brand. So why don't you come in, if we offer you a 10 percent discount for the next hour? See how enticing this offer is? This marketing experience is much more targeted and precise, therefore has a better chance of being actually successful.

We already see some mobile applications changing these behavior patterns. Aviate has been getting attention for their rethinking of the mobile home screen, which changes as you go with your day. When you wake up, it highlights relevant morning functionalities such as weather and calendar and changes later depending on activities. **The idea of a mobile device reacting to our lifestyle without the need to search and activate each function is where the future is.**

Dating is one of the first verticals killing the search function. By using GPS technology, mobile startups such as SinglesAroundMe and MeetMoi connect strangers on the go, as they live their lives and walk on the streets of their neighborhoods. Right now, they are powered by instant human connection—when you see someone you like, you send a signal and connect. But what if the device was actually signaling you when you walk by someone who could be a good match with?

The same approach is already used for content recommendations. Instead of scanning newspapers, magazines, RSS feeds, blogs and Twitter streams, only to find a fraction of the content matching our interests, we have the best matches delivered to us by services like News.me. I start my morning with its daily e-mail delivering important articles to me that my social circle is buzzing about, and it rarely misses.

The content discovery is also happening on social platforms like Facebook and Twitter, where we get content recommendations from our friends and followers. In addition to providing an instant personalization, these networks are turning all of us into instant curators or editors of content.

Assuming that you've built a network of people with similar interests, you may never have to search for content again. You can simply rely on your network to deliver the top news to you, or point you in the right direction when visiting your favorite destinations.

Of course, this system still requires someone to discover and share content in the first place, and search is one of the ways to do so. But it's only a matter of time until new technologies fill in the gaps left by your network, and ensure you receive every piece of relevant content from across the web, prioritized accordingly.

With successful adaptation of personalized recommendations in the content consumption area, suggestions are becoming one of the

main drivers of online shopping. Right now they are heavily based on friends and social networks; however, future technologies will allow live auto-suggestions being offered on the go.

If you've ever tried searching for an item of clothing or an accessory, you probably got lost in thousands of product choices, only a fraction of which would suit your needs. What if new clothes were selectively offered to you, based on your characteristics, taste and budget as they come into stores?

Even today, universal social platforms like Facebook are able to provide enough personal data for a variety of technologies to automate these common processes, essentially replacing our need to search.

It's not a coincidence that Facebook has begun to surpass Google as the most visited site in the U.S. The shift will continue as we change our behavior from searching for things to discovering things through our social networks and geo-location services.

Seasons Are So Last Season.

As fashion industry continues to evolve and becomes more digitized, the old rules will have to change. Collections, seasons, fashion weeks, buyers, magazine editors—everything and everyone are being challenged these days. Inevitably, many processes will be redefined, and powers will shift.

Despite the threat to the old-school industry establishments, the restructure will be a healthy thing and will eventually lead to enhanced productivity, which in turn will leave fashion brands and retailers with more time and resources to innovate. One of the reasons that fashion brands don't heavily invest in innovation is that they're preoccupied with the chase after the next season.

Most brands currently operate in an endless loop, producing two to eight collections every year, which leaves them no time to pause, look around, notice the ways the world is changing and come up with a strategy that suits this change. It is hard to pause when they have clients, buyers, manufacturers and a schedule to keep up with, but this way of operating won't be sustainable in the long term.

The chase after Spring, Fall, Resort and Pre-Fall seasons is pointless when we have chains like H&M and Target coming up with collections every week or so. What's interesting about these collections is the fact that they often cross the lines between seasons, and their pieces could be mixed and matched. Examples: Jimmy Choo for H&M, Rodarte and Zac Posen for Target—all included dresses that could be worn both during summer and winter, not to mention open-toe sandals sold by H&M in December.

How can an average brand compete with these chains pushing all kinds of products continuously year-round? Following the rules and designing collections by seasons might not make much sense in this fast-paced environment. Although the way we dress is still influenced by the weather outside, our shopping habits don't always reflect that. People travel the globe more than ever, and changing climate zones isn't a novelty anymore. Of course, the clothes themselves are still seasonal by nature, but that doesn't mean designers have to introduce them all at the same time, twice a year during their regional fashion week, and then later launch at the same time in the same retail locations, like a department store.

Another limitation is the full collections that designers are forcing themselves to produce each season. Most of these collections consist of basics, which don't change much from season to season, and trendy staple pieces, which change according to seasonal trends. It's not efficient to start every season from scratch, creating basics and staple pieces. Sportswear companies are a great example to a more effective approach. Take Adidas, which has the same basic sneakers available from year to year, and releases special limited-edition themed sneakers a few times a year.

Fashion designers could adopt similar approach and keep their bestselling basics from season to season, saving on production. This will also allow them to focus their energy on the most creative items, which truly express who they are. In addition, just like people who buy fewer music albums and instead purchase individual songs on iTunes, consumers today are not necessarily shopping for the entire look from the same brand, but rather are looking for a single special piece to add to their wardrobe.

Designers should be focusing on creating bestselling pieces which can stand out on their own, instead of worrying about making a cohesive seasonal collection to please fashion critics.

Online retailers like Net-A-Porter already are experimenting in this direction of smaller item-focused collections, by inviting designers like Roland Mouret, who launched six limited-edition mini dresses with the e-tailer in 2011.

Another great example of a brand that focused on making one basic item a bestselling piece and even came up with an entirely separate branding for it is DKNY and its signature Cozy wrap cardigan. It's so popular that it has its own app, in which people can learn about different ways to wear it. Each season the Cozy gets a slight upgrade or special edition, but the basic idea stays the same. This allows the brand to create longevity and extend the success of one product through the years.

Diane Von Furstenberg's signature wrap dress is another staple product that gets an update through the years, but has been a true bestseller for decades now.

More designers should be creating products with long-term goals and thinking about turning them into multi-seasonal successes, instead of trying to capture the current trend of the season and move onto something else in the next collection. Only a long-term approach could create truly innovative products.

There is something liberating about the idea of ignoring seasons and focusing only on great products. Of course you may say that not every brand has the luxury to do so—that they depend on buyers who work by certain schedules and department stores which move merchandise based on certain plans.

This is where the beauty of online retail comes in again. There is no need to follow rules—the online customers are coming from all over the world, from different climates and different demographics. Every item created has a potential to reach its target consumer at any given time. **While department stores have to answer to the local demand, online stores have limitless possibilities when it comes to reaching the right customer.**

The true change will happen once designers recognize this opportunity and start catering to the online customer when it comes to collections, seasons and items they produce.

We often look up to the consumers' electronics industry as the most forward-thinking. Releases like the iPad shake up the media and our wallets, and often even change our life. I believe the clothing and footwear industry has the same potential to create buzz around new releases once they stop chasing after the old rules of releasing full-blown collections twice a year.

Imagine if Apple had to replace their entire inventory twice a year, releasing all-new collection of iPads, iPods, notebooks, desktops and screens every fall and spring. Will they be able to innovate the same way they do now? Sure, they do upgrade their products and release new versions every so often, but if you look at the entire year you will notice only one or two revolutionary releases that change the market, and sometimes our lives.

What if fashion designers or brands focused on revolutionizing our lives instead of chasing after trends someone defines for them? What if they invested their creativity in solving our everyday wardrobe problems? I believe this industry is just at the beginning of reaching its potential as something life-changing and revolutionary. There is no reason our clothes won't be as functional and durable as some of the gadgets we covet.

If there is anything fashion brands can learn from iPad, it is the fact that even today consumers are willing to pay $700 for a product that is well made and life-changing. And if people are willing to pay

$700 for a sexy gadget that does the same thing every desktop does, they will be willing to pay that price for an innovative item of clothing they will be wearing for years, regardless of seasons and trends.

Another thing they can learn is that Apple has put lots of thought into the iPad. Is it worth investing the same effort in a dress, you might ask. If this dress could be the universal must-have dress for millions of people, I think it is well worth it. If these smart shoes will shorten the commute time for millions of people, I think it is.

So why are designers, instead of focusing on one best seller, one product that they will be remembered for, so caught up in the endless cycle of sketching, producing, styling, bowing on the runway, pleasing buyers, gifting celebs, spoiling press, praying for it all to pay off, and then repeating over and over every season?

Why not adopt the consumer electronics model and focus on creating a fashionable item so covetable that when it launches the entire world wants a piece of it?

How about, instead of sending ten coats down the runway, a designer or brand focuses on one coat that is multifunctional, can address multiple climate needs and easily change appearance? A coat that will replace all the other coats a person ever owned because they won't live up to the standard? It doesn't mean everyone should be wearing the same coat from now on. It can still come in different fabrics and variations, but the product itself must be innovative in order to become the iPad of fashion.

Trends are for Masses,
Personal Style is for Individuals.

Just like with seasons, trends are losing their value in the fast paced, innovation-driven age. The natural cycle of a trend — early adoption, mainstream recognition and finally mass consumption — is getting so short, that it challenges the concept itself.

On any given day at a store like H&M, you can see twenty different time-period influences and countless cultural references. The eclectic style that was widely adopted by bloggers and street style photographers is pushing the fashion limits and introduces a new trend: personal style.

Of course, people with distinctive personal style always existed in any society, but today the idea of having unique point of view is encouraged and celebrated. The ability to stylishly mix a vintage jacket with a pair of latest hot denim brand and a Kmart T-shirt is admired. Magazines dedicate spreads to high-and-low, mix-and-match fashion and educate consumers on the different ways to create their wardrobe with new and old items.

There is no right and wrong in today's fashion — it's all about the confidence with which you carry your style. Current trends carry less and less weight. Personal style is the hot new commodity.

What does this mean for designers and brands? Unfortunately, this means they can't rely on trends anymore. Trend forecasting agencies are still in the market and influence what we see on the racks, but their role will continue to diminish as democratization of fashion trends continue to grow.

Today designers get inspired by street-style photography from Japan posted online almost in real time, they get inspired by consumers styling items their own way and posting it on their Instagram accounts. The process is a two-way street, versus a top-down trend dictation.

The challenge for designers is a tough one—instead of simply following trend forecasting reports, spicing them up with unique points of view and delivering collections, they now have to cater to the highly personalized style trend, which is unique to everyone. How can they personally cater to a 25-year-old mom in Alabama and a 25-year-old career girl in New York City?

Brands still lack sophisticated tools to study and analyze consumers, which is partially the reason for this disconnect. Digital technologies now allow retailers to study consumer demand and behavior via their e-commerce sites. They can get live response on their products via social media. This is a huge advantage that brands haven't had in the past. They had to use forecasting tools and estimates in order to predict consumer behavior and they wouldn't know the results until the product hit the stores. Think about the high risk of this operation. This is the biggest gamble of the fashion industry, the industry that is leaving retailers with millions of unwanted clothes on the racks every season.

Today brands could potentially get the idea of product demand from the moment the clothes are shown on the runway. High amount of Facebook "likes" on a particular dress can indicate potential retail demand and help brands optimize their production cycles.

In addition to getting insights into consumer behavior the biggest advantage digital technology is giving the brands is the ability to know the consumer in a way they could never before. Between the Facebook Connect platform and e-commerce accounts, the amount of data stored online on each person is incredible. Accessing and analyzing this data gives every e-tailer a chance to get to know their customers on a personal level. This gives them the ability to customize offers based on personality, demographics, lifestyle and more. And customers can discover only products they love and not waste time looking at something they could never afford or something they would never be interested in.

For example, currently visiting Saks.com, every visitor—male or female, old or young—is seeing the exact same homepage. It usually features a few looks based on the trends defined by brand merchandisers. It has nothing to do with the person visiting the store. A person who dislikes pink and would never wear it may be still presented with a pink jacket on Saks.com homepage. What a waste! Imagine the possibilities if Saks.com used profile data to show shoppers only items with high purchase potential.

Amazon has been on the forefront of e-commerce innovation with its personalized recommendations. It clearly didn't build an empire just by bringing thousands of retailers together. It built its empire by studying its customers and delivering what they want.

Truly smart personalized shopping is still ahead of us, but is surely coming. Once we overcome the fear of sharing private information online and become less sensitive to the blurring line of private versus public, we will see innovation flourish. This will profoundly change our online experience. By opening up, we can discover new things, whether it's news, products or people.

Trends will become less relevant. What would truly matter: How does a particular product make you look, feel, and behave? How does it affect your personality and how does it fit into your lifestyle— whether it's last year's trend or a vintage piece from forty years ago?

Retailers that focus on consumer needs and taste instead of seeking industry approval will eventually win.

If You Could Have Fashion Week Year-Round, Why Wouldn't You?

Now that we looked at the decreasing importance of seasonal collections and trends, the question is this: What is the purpose of the seasonal fashion weeks, in which trends are defined and collections are bought?

These days, runway shows are slowly turning into marketing platforms for brands. They are transforming from insider-only events attended mainly by magazine editors and buyers into highly publicized events syndicated live across multiple channels.

However there is still confusion about who these fashion shows are staged for. Right now, many of them are attended by buyers, editors, online press, celebrities, important customers and people at home who watch them live on their computer screens. Each group of people watches the show for different reasons; however, more designers are staging to focus on entertainment, décor and spectacle, targeting masses over industry insiders. After all, having a bigger audience helps to justify the high cost of their investments in such events.

These events are not able to fully capitalize on the buzz, however, since the items shown are not yet available for purchase. There is no call to action, and no return on investment. This missed opportunity will have to be resolved to bring more efficiency into the industry.

Perhaps we could learn from Melbourne Fashion Festival, Australia's largest public consumer and retail-driven fashion event. Pieces shown on Melbourne runways are available for immediate purchase, making the shows an effective marketing tool. In addition, there is an industry-only fashion week in Sydney, Australia that focuses on buyers, agents, stylists and other industry representatives.

In 2012, when visiting Magic—the biggest retail conference and trade show in Las Vegas—I was surprised to see a huge space full of fashion brands, each with their own booth and a representative equipped with line sheets and paper forms for potential buyers. It was hard to believe that the majority of the buying business was still done on the trade show floor on pieces of paper. After I gave my keynote talk on social media trends and the way they are changing fashion, several people approached me and said they wished their boss/designer/buyer were more aware of the things I was talking about. At Magic I felt transported to a time before computers entered our life.

As technology progresses and learns to capture the reality in an easier way, the buying process will become completely digitized. This is one of the biggest inefficiencies in the industry that several startups, Joor among them, are trying to solve.

Major challenges in this space include connecting designers and buyers, streamlining orders, and managing inventory. All these can be easily solved with cloud computing. Of course you might argue that buyers still need to see the clothes in person, and that no computer screen can replace the touch of a fabric, but the more that shoppers move online and trust their computer screens to pick their latest fashions, the more it proves that buyers could use a similar but better-equipped system.

Startups like MIKA are experimenting with the ways that garments are presented online by incorporating movement and bringing still image to life. Video is becoming a common component on many e-commerce sites, with Zappos and Yoox leading the way.

In addition, the role and importance of a buyer is challenged by the growing trend of brands adopting direct e-commerce. It's been easier than ever for any brand to open a sophisticated online store, with lots of functionalities and data. They don't have to rely on buyers and retailers anymore in order to reach customers. Direct e-commerce is a powerful channel for a brand's marketing and sales.

In a world in which people discover products on Pinterest or search for items on ShopStyle, there is less importance to a retailer like Macy's curating the inventory. Brands are becoming more independent from buyers' opinions, they can test and release products directly to consumers.

This is where an event like Fashion Week, targeted at consumers, can really close the loop. If a brand is in charge of showing and selling collections, why would it be dependent on someone else's schedule and opinion? With today's mass technology, every brand has the ability to show product, syndicate content to millions of consumers via social media, and instantly sell product via direct e-commerce channels. They can control the entire process and take full advantage of it, unlike in the past, when they had to rely on magazine editors for syndication and on retail buyers for sales.

Think about this shift in power for a moment. **Brands today are fully in charge of their success. They can create their own rules, yet they choose to follow the old ones.** They create collections to please the buyers and they choose to show them along with their peers during the designated fashion week times. Inertion law? Probably. How long will things continue moving in the same direction? Not for long, I predict. Brands need to wake up and realize there are no more limits, that nothing that can hold them back and control their destiny. They have to start making their own rules—whether they choose to present a full collection or just one dress, whether they do it in September or January, and whether they're competing with hundreds of their peers at fashion week events.

Once brands release themselves of these mental limitations, the possibilities for introducing their products will be endless. Maybe it's a runway show, an art installation or a concert? Perhaps it's an ongoing event released in parts, just like a TV series, driving anticipation? Maybe it's part crowd-sourced? The new product presentation can be anything, not just an expensive five-minute-long runway show in which people fight for the best iPhone shot from the last row.

CHAPTER FOUR:
PRODUCT

Compared to other industries, fashion is still very low-tech, and mostly relies on inventions of the past centuries: the sewing machine, artificial dyes, zippers, stitching, etc. The only things that have been changing are the shapes of our clothes and the processes in which they are made and sold. With the digitization of our clothes, the possibilities are endless.

On Fashion and Singularity.

The past two decades were all about new electronic devices. We were introduced to desktop computers, then laptops, digital music players and smartphones, all helping us to power and navigate through our lives. These devices have been slowly taking over some of the basic functions of our brains, allowing us to focus on creative and sophisticated tasks.

These devices have been exponentially decreasing in size and increasing in their abilities. They have also become more flexible in form and shape.

We are already seeing experiments with different interfaces that replace the need for the screen-based devices which most of us use today to connect to the internet. This technology allows fabrics and other surfaces to act as screens—or even the devices themselves.

The new emerging trend is M2M (Machine-to-Machine), in which previously "dumb" everyday objects will become increasingly connected to the web. Everything will have the capacity to become "smart."

Also enabling these new devices is the growing Wi-Fi infrastructure, which eventually will connect pretty much every single point on earth. As technology becomes less expensive, we will become less constricted with wireless providers and various devices.

In the near future, we will be able to connect wirelessly from anywhere and with any type of device. Eventually, devices will play less important role, as different objects and surfaces develop the ability to connect. In the long term, even our physical body will have the ability to connect. This will turn us, humans, into the most powerful devices to date. This point of time is known as Singularity.

For those new to the concept, *"The Singularity represents an 'event horizon' in the predictability of human technological development past which present models of the future may cease to give reliable answers, following the creation of strong Artificial Intelligence or the enhancement of human intelligence."*

According to Ray Kurzweil, one of the leading inventors of our times, the paradigm shift rate is now doubling every decade, and eventually the pace of technological change will be so rapid, its impact so deep, that human life will be irreversibly transformed.

In his book *The Singularity Is Near*, published in 2005, Kurzweil predicts, among other things, that by 2020, personal computers will have the same processing power as human brains, and soon after computers less than 100 nm (0.0001mm) in size will be possible.

Of course, this statement may scare older people, who once listened to cassette tapes and wrote letters to each other. Unfortunately, the exponentially developing technology will reach that point earlier than most human beings are willing to actually adopt it. It might take a completely digitally raised generation of people to fully embrace the technological capabilities of the next decade.

This means there will be a transitional period in which people are willing to take advantage of the Artificial Intelligence and smart devices guiding them through life, but not willing to have them embedded in their bodies … yet.

Wearable devices will emerge during this period. We are at the tipping point at which wearable devices will reach mass markets. What does this mean for clothing and accessories brands and retailers? A whole new era of new, smart, interactive, experimental clothing.

In the process in which machines are becoming part of our bodies, clothes will play an important role and serve as an interim phase. As comfortable as people are with plastic surgeries, and the implanting of hearing aids and peacemakers, installing wireless devices in their bodies will require much more of an open mind. This is where the clothes come in. In the phase of our cyborg transformation, the clothes—our second skin—will play a crucial part in seamlessly connecting us from any place at any point in time. They will be the device *and* the interface.

Holy Nike, My Shoes are Tweeting.

There is a huge future for the "wearable computing" built into our clothing. The first development we've been seeing on the road to smart clothing is **wired clothing,** mostly explored so far by sport apparel companies such as Nike and Burton, and the health industry for monitoring heart rate.

One example is a SmartShirt, which monitors biometric information in an easy and wearable manner. The electrical fibers woven into the shirt can detect and record heart rate, body temperature, heat rates and calories burned. This information can be shared with the wearer via the embedded microphone, or sent wirelessly to a doctor or coach. A variety of companies have been developing their version of smart shirts, with VivoMetrics claiming the first commercial product.

Besides smart shirts, each item in our wardrobe has the potential to become an electronic surface or a platform for various apps and devices. Just like our laptops come with USB ports, our clothes of the future could have such ports embedded in the buttons. This will allow any garment to have functionalities beyond fashion. Our clothes will be much more valuable and people will be willing to pay higher prices for even basic "smart" garments.

But first, we will see a variety of fashion accessories turning digital. A few are already hitting the market. Right now these devices are not designed with a fashion consumer in mind; however, they have a huge potential to replace "dumb" accessories—bracelets, rings, glasses—that serve no purpose other than visual.

For example, the MYO gesture control armband lets its wearer use the electrical activity in his muscles to wirelessly control a computer, phone, and his other favorite digital technologies. Incorporating this into a trendy silver bracelet would create a multi-functional, covetable product.

Google's Project Glass allows people to get the full online experience on their glasses. Now Google is looking to collaborate with the trendy startup Warby Parker to make the glasses not only a smart device, but a desirable fashion accessory.

Accessories are the most natural and easiest objects to turn digital. For example, jewelry already contains metals, so, more than fabrics, it could more easily accommodate integrated electronics. Smart watches are already a reality and now designers are experimenting with Bluetooth earrings and more technologically advanced wearable accessories.

Telepathy One, a headpiece developed by Japanese inventor Takahito Iguchi, allows a wearer to share his picture with any of his friends without touching a device. The founders chose to focus on the design aspects from day one, realizing the importance of visual appearance when it comes to smart wearable devices made for mass market. While Google Glass's approach is to bring the entire smartphone experience into your eye, Telepathy One has more of an iPod approach—it focuses on one function only and perfects it. A wearer can take an instant photo through a simple voice command and share it wirelessly on their social networks. The social sharing aspect is the most obvious use for a device that lets other people see through your eyes.

Another fashion-tech Google project is being done in collaboration with Adidas and artist Zach Lieberman. With interactive collective YesYesNO, they are creating a smart Adidas sneaker that can talk and share the owner's activity on the web. The shoe works as a fitness-tracking device using an accelerometer, Bluetooth and other technologies to analyze the wearer's movements. This project wasn't made for retail production, but just as an art piece; however, adapting the same concept for retail is only a matter of time.

Microsoft has also joined the wearable-devices race. With its Wearable Multitouch Projector, a brooch or lapel pin could turn any surface into an interactive display. Imagine walking down the street and projecting GPS directions on the sidewalk. This projector still needs a mobile phone to work, but as our devices become smaller eventually there won't be a need to have a phone as our main device connecting us online.

GraphExeter, a material produced by a team from the University's Centre for Graphene Science, is made of grapheme—the most transparent, lightweight and flexible material ever invented for conducting electricity. The material, just a few atoms thick, is flexible and strong. As a conductor of electricity, it performs as well as copper; and as a conductor of heat, it outperforms all other known materials. This means it could be used to make clothing containing computers and other electronic equipment.

Another interesting development may completely eliminate the need for seasonal clothes. Body temperature balancing clothes could potentially turn a thin T-shirt into a garment as warm as a cashmere sweater. Our body's temperature naturally changes throughout the day, so why shouldn't our clothing? Outlast Adaptive Comfort products store excess heat as it's created and release it as it's needed, so you can do labor-intensive activities longer. Nano-Tex Coolest Comfort gives wearers the freedom to move from hot to cold environments and still feel dry, all day long. Its advanced moisture wicking keeps wearers cool without changing the way their clothes feel.

These exciting inventions are just the first signs of a new era of fashion innovations. Our clothing, which hasn't been updated much for the past century beyond shapes and trendy looks, is finally getting some serious interest from scientists and inventors. I can't wait to see what they come up with. Heels that make you walk two times faster? A universal dress that comes with a fabric-changing app? Or a body-cooling statement necklace for the summer season? There is so much room for invention!

Fabrics are Getting Smarter.

The inventions described in the earlier chapter might sound futuristic, considering how low-tech our clothes still are. Yes, most of them are still considered disposable items, something that you buy every season or so and pray for it to last through ten laundry cycles. Advancing the materials is the key to fashion innovation and digitization of this industry. After all, we can't build a sophisticated interactive experience on such low-tech canvases as cotton, leather and silk.

The fabrics have to become smart, just like our phones slowly became smart. They have to become digital canvases, merging online innovation with our second skins—our clothes. Several new developments aim to help our clothes become the durable, long-lasting item it needs to be to justify digital integrations.

Let's start with smart cleaning. Laundry machines definitely made our lives easier, but they still require special installation, access to water and multiple products like detergents, bleachers and softeners to do the job. After all this effort they may still ruin the fabric, especially in the long run. Wouldn't it be great to come up with an alternative?

The Naturewash by Zhenpeng Li is a true futuristic laundry system. It's a waterless washer that cleans nano-coated fabric clothes using negative ions. Imagine simply spreading your clothes on the machine surface to get rid of dirt.

Drying is another issue. Instantly dry clothes could eliminate the need for drying time. For example, swimwear that dries itself instantly is not a dream anymore, thanks to Sun Dry Swim, which features quick-dry nanotechnology enhanced swimwear fabric that sheds water as naturally as skin. It's only a matter of time until this technology will make it into apparel, making the rainy days much less wet and eliminating the need for driers.

A newly released NeverWet spray completely repels water and heavy oils. Any object coated with it, even a pair of white canvas sneakers, literally cannot be touched by liquid. Any liquid placed on this coating is repelled and magically rolls off without touching the underlying surface, basically eliminating the need for laundry or dry cleaning.

One reason for frequent clothes-washes is to eliminate odors. What if our clothes didn't absorb odors? Japanese company Teijin, known for applying cutting-edge technologies to textiles, has developed a range of solutions, including anti-bacterial odor prevention.

Carnation Footcare has launched silver-lined socks that keep feet warm and smelling of roses—or so it claims. Pure silver, which coats the outside of the textile fibers, kills bacteria and neutralizes bad odor-causing elements.

Of course staining is still the number-one destroyer of clothing. There are plenty of stain removers on the market today, but what if the fabric itself wasn't even able to catch stains? Nano-Tex, a fabric innovation company providing textile enhancements to the apparel market, recently rolled out the market's best-performing stain repel-and-release treatment. The new solution could eliminate the need for the most innovative stain remover.

Next challenge: keeping clothes perfectly ironed and crisp-looking. The process of ironing did improve their appearance, but it's tedious and doesn't produce a long-lasting effect. A new technique allows the garments to be treated with an anti-wrinkle finish before the garment is dyed. This chemical treatment minimizes wrinkles and gives a smooth appearance to the fabrics. Hopefully, the days of heavy ironing will be soon over.

Mass adoption of these materials would be crucial to the advancement of our clothes and becoming more "smart." Just like electronic devices are expected to possess durability, our clothes need to get there as well to become a real interface for digital innovation.

Dressing in a Push of a Button.

Once our fabrics become digitized, they could contain and transmit data, be controlled by devices, and merge the online and offline experience by becoming the interface. From there, the possibilities would be endless.

Many futuristic developments are already being developed in labs and are being tested by innovative companies all over the world. These companies are having a hard time integrating into mass retail, however—mostly because of the high cost of these materials and partially because of the unwillingness or inability of fashion brands to invest resources and time in exploring and testing the innovations. One day, however, the need to develop a competitive edge will force brands to get into the lab, or risk staying irrelevant.

Many fashion brands didn't believe in the importance of social media and refused to allocate resources to it—until they couldn't avoid the fact that having a social presence is a must, not a luxury. Digital materials are next. They are about to introduce a whole new world to the designers, creating a new digital playground for these creative people. Let's look at some of the most exciting innovations to enter our lives.

One of the latest inventions in the field of light-emitting devices might change the way clothes are designed: color changing clothes.

The device, currently being developed by a consortium of scientists from six different countries called Modecom, represents a thin film of plastic able to conduct electricity. Because organic light-emitting devices are thin and flexible, electronic display screens could be easily created on nearly every material. Thus, for example, clothing could for the first time in history display specific electronic information. There are various ways of using the OLED; for example, it could be used to change the color of clothes.

As a result, the idea of trend and color forecasting, which dictates the seasonal looks today, could be challenged. There will be simply no need to predict color palettes. The consumer would be in charge of choosing colors from the menu or patterns from the available library. Designers and brands won't need to produce the same garment in multiple colors and department store buyers won't have to guess what would sell better—a black cardigan or a blue one. Finally, consumers could invest in one product and get the most out of having multiple colors available in just one push of a button.

In addition, this invention will also reduce waste—instead of buying multiple colors of the same garment, we will be able to purchase one and change it according to our mood or occasion.

Another important invention relates to the shape of our clothes. Perhaps the "Airplane dress" that Hussein Chalayan created as part of his 2000 spring collection looked too futuristic, but the concept itself of shape-changing clothes isn't as far from our reality. Imagine a skirt that could change from an A-line to pencil shape in a click of a button. Just as with color, garments can become a long-lasting, multi-functional investment, rather than the disposable low-tech objects they are today.

The trend of convertible clothing isn't new. We are seeing designers today experimenting with garments you can wear several ways, dresses that become skirts, coats that become jackets, two-sided garments—the opportunities for innovative multi-functional garments are endless. By adding a digital layer, we could potentially have an all-in-one garment that changes color and shape based on our needs.

Once fabrics become more sophisticated and shapes are controlled, sizing and fitting—the main reason people spend so much time shopping, trying things on, returning merchandise and replacing items after slight weight fluctuation—may no longer be an issue. If only our clothes could adjust to our changes in body shape, all of this could be resolved. Size-adjustable clothes have yet to be invented, but they have the potential to change the fashion world as they would solve the biggest problem in mass clothing manufacturing—the unique shape of each human body. Size-adjustable shoes are today's reality, thanks to INCHworm, although they haven't yet seen huge market penetration. Imagine what size-adjustable clothes could do!

While it'll take some time to get our clothes fully adjustable, the transition will bring lots of innovative concepts. One: interchangeable parts with a multi-functional base. OneSole is an example of a shoe with interchangeable tops that could be attached to the same sole. This concept could be also applied to clothing and other accessories.

Lastly, one of the biggest innovations in clothing production is the 3-D printing, which is slowly penetrating into mass consumption. Jewelry was the first category to jump on the trend, with emerging designers creating an entire brand around 3-D printed pieces. As 3-D printers reach the consumers and become as affordable as personal paper printers, everyone will be turning into a designer and a production house, all in one. Of course making one's own clothes isn't for everyone, but I believe more people will experiment with production, and that will significantly lower the barrier to entry for new designers and brands.

It will also open a new category of companies that create templates for clothes and accessories, to be printed by consumers at home. The trend has already started with furniture and design objects, with Ponoco pioneering the market. Fashion is the next natural choice. Companies like Shapeways create marketplaces for people to buy and sell 3-D products, introducing the concept to the masses.

These ideas might sounds too futuristic for mass market integration, but with the decreased costs of new technologies they will become standard in apparel industry in the next few years. Pressured by the economy, fashion designers and brands are so busy these days thinking about the next season—at a time they should be thinking about the next decade. If our clothes could be compared to computers, we are still wearing DOS. It's time for an overall system upgrade.

CHAPTER FIVE:

LIFESTYLE

In earlier chapters, we talked about the effects of the digital revolution on consumers, brands, retailers, and products. The next and final chapter is dedicated to the change in our lifestyle—from our bodies to the way we power them, and use them to interact and consume.

The Digitization of our Bodies.

The digital revolution we've been seeing so far has mostly affected our minds. It created a new dimension, in which many of us are spending a big part of our lives socially connected through various networks, apps and devices. Many of our brain tasks are now done by computers, and lots of our memories are stored in the digital cloud. Our social connections are managed by computers as well, allowing us to interact, create, and even feel.

However, our bodies are still disconnected from that virtual world. I believe the anxiety many of us feel towards the new technology is rooted in this disconnect. The digital life seems like another dimension that distracts us from the real life, its pleasures and experiences. People go on digital detoxes and try to limit the time they spend online, as if it were an unhealthy habit. The digital world may seem unnatural because our body is disconnected from it, so it's not perceived as part of human nature.

This may change once technology becomes part of our bodies, and is seamlessly integrated into them. Much of what we do at the computer, we will be doing while walking, talking or even sleeping. Mobile phones are the first step towards the digital experience on the go. Google Glasses and other wearable technologies are the next step, and finally chips implanted into our bodies and connected directly to our brains will finish our transition into the powerful next generation of human beings—cyborgs, Human Body 2.0, whatever you choose to call it.

Back in 2003, Ray Kurzweil wrote that "in the coming decades, a radical upgrading of our body's physical and mental systems, already underway, will use nanobots to augment and ultimately replace our organs. By 2030, reverse-engineering of the human brain will have been completed and nonbiological intelligence will merge with our biological brains."

Today in 2013, with all the technological progress we've made in the past decade, this radical thought is still difficult to digest. It is important to understand the bigger revolution that's happening around us, however, to prepare ourselves for the next decade.

I find this transition to be most fascinating of all, and feel lucky to witness it as an adult who was born in a completely analog world and will probably leave this world when it's completely digitized. Not many generations have the opportunity to witness such a transformational and enlightening experience.

Let's see what this change will transform the fashion industry.

Meet the Virtual Instance of Your Body.

One of the transition points in our own human digitization process is creating a virtual version of our bodies. This version mimics our physical body in shape and size and allows us to test products, track results and analyze data about our activities.

For example, health and fitness apps help us optimize our lifestyle and track our progress based on our virtual profiles.

In fashion, smart technologies allow us to virtually try on clothes and optimize our looks, saving real-life trial and error. They translate our bodies into virtual avatars and create an entirely new playground for brands. From virtual hair and makeup tools to virtual dressing rooms, testing products on our virtual bodies is becoming part of the consuming process.

The 3-D virtual-body technologies haven't yet become adopted by the masses; however, a large number of companies have been creating products to accelerate that.

Online retail companies like MyShape, Fits.me and UpCload are working on integrating with mass retailers to introduce the virtual body idea into our shopping experience.

The virtual bodies of our times don't necessarily have to be a 3-D version of our human self, just like Second Life tried to do back in

2003 by building a 3-D replica of our reality. Our body doesn't need to be translated so literally. A virtual instance, such as mobile app storing data about your body and its health, is sufficient to provide the same results. In a similar way, a fashion app that stores your shape data based on the measurements of your webcam creates another instance of your virtual body.

These instances make up our virtual ID and eventually will allow for the deep personalization of our online experience, including the way we discover and shop for products.

The matchmaking between people and products will eventually be done on the go, based on these profiles and without much human interaction.

Clothes will be perfectly matched to your body and products will be recommended based on your lifestyle, without us having to fill out long forms and play "yes" or "no" games to help an application learn your taste.

With time, our digital profiles will become so rich and sophisticated, the data collected over years so robust, that our entire life experience can be planned by computers without much effort on our part.

Our Life Tracked and Optimized.

Now that we have apps that have a version of our virtual body and collect data about its different activities, we can optimize our life in multitude of ways. What we are seeing now is only the beginning of this process, as we've been just busy collecting data for the past decade. We now have online data on the ways we exercise, eat, work, shop, and even sleep.

What do we do with all this data? The next step in this evolution is to learn how to use it to make our lives more productive and tailored to us. This affects every aspect of our lives.

In marketing, we are seeing a major shift from top-down advertising to integrated marketing and now adaptive marketing. It means that advertising is no longer pushed to us at the most inconvenient time, promoting products least relevant to our lifestyles. Advertising is actually becoming helpful in the discovery of new products and solutions.

There is a new term that brands are starting to reference—adaptive marketing. It includes promotions that are offered as a reaction on person's daily activities, suggesting the most relevant services and products.

Apps like Foursquare or products like Google Glass are most likely to introduce this concept into masses, since these platforms are built for seamless integration on the go. A person walking by a clothing store may get recommendations based on his or her style and fit, without even walking through the door.

The world will evolve around our desires and preferences, serving us our favorite things instead of us hunting for them. Sure, there is a pleasure in the hunt—but, if you could take the time you wasted trying on a hundred pairs of jeans just to find one that flatters, and spent it on more valuable things, you would receive a deeper and long-lasting form of satisfaction.

"Optimizing our lifestyle" is the new slogan of our decade and it's going to be a fascinating time, especially for those who remember the challenges of the analog world. Streamlining the bureaucratic, inefficient processes that currently fill our life will allow all of us as a society to focus on things that matter.

In the Age of Information, Data is the New Retail Currency.

While our technologies collect millions of data points for every individual, their taste, body shape and lifestyle, we don't see much of this data being used in retail. It is still surprising that today, with so much information publicly available through various platforms, most retailers opt to present their online customers with the same non-personalized web experience.

Several e-commerce-enhancing tools are starting to offer a personalization layer. Technology available today is capable of customizing an experience for each customer without much investment on retailers' side. This will not only improve sales conversion, but save time to shoppers that would have been wasted on searching and browsing through thousands of irrelevant products.

The way we catalog and offer products will have to change as the online supply and choices grow. With millions of empowered individuals joining the marketplace and offering their own products—in addition to established retailers increasing their offerings—we are close to a point at which both search and discovery are becoming challenging for the average consumer. Too many offerings become a negative; they'll turn people away from online shopping.

Curation has been the buzzword of the past few years; however, the manual element involved in curation doesn't allow for significant scale. Scale is the main reason that I believe data analysts will be the merchandisers of the future. The only way to sort through millions of product offerings, categorize them in a meaningful way, and match them successfully with interested consumers will be through the analytical tools of the future.

Matchmaking products and consumers is the toughest challenge of the decade that machines can't solve yet. As they become smarter, however, they will learn human behavioral patterns and will be able to make the right choices for us. This will change online retailing forever. Instead of replicating physical stores in online dimension, like we are seeing today, we will be seeing online platforms that study our lifestyles and offer relevant options from the endless pool of choices.

Amazon is one of the first retailers to realize the future and build a robust platform that relies less on its own brand and its curators than on smart cataloging and its recommendation engine. It is the company to watch for revolutionizing fashion shopping experience online, even though many might not perceive it as their go-to source… yet. The data that Amazon is already collecting about our shopping habits and lifestyle, crossed with the enormous pool of retailers and product choices they offer, will be powerful when it comes to the future of retail.

Just like online tracking tools that analyze online shoppers' behavior, mobile technologies are bringing the data layer to the physical stores. Retailers like C.Wonder are experimenting with active RFID chips embedded into items to track their performance. By following the movement patterns of the products throughout the store—from storage to fitting rooms to cashiers—the retailer can learn and optimize store signage, merchandizing and offers.

Another way to track consumers and offer promotions is through location-based mobile technologies and user check-ins. One company competing in the personalized retail offers space is ShopKick. It relies on customers' existing mobile phones to track their experience and offer rewards. In this case, the main implementation is done on the retailer's side—ShopKick installs devices in-store, similar to Wi-Fi access points, and the device sends inaudible audio signals, which interact with a phone's microphone. The offers, which include the ability to earn points, Facebook currency, song downloads, and instant gift cards that can be redeemed in-store, get sent to the phone.

These new tools connect retailers and consumers in the physical store environment, allowing virtual data access from the moment someone walks into the store. Even though the image of a personal shopper greeting you at the entrance by name and offering you clothes in your size and your favorite color feels like a Big Brother experience to most of us, the convenience will eventually outweigh the fear.

As we get used to the fact that our information is shared in order to optimize our lives, it will open a creative playground for brands. It will allow them to tailor unique experiences to individuals instead of catering to the average masses, as they do today. The idea of mass retail may even disappear. As brands get smarter with the ways they use data and treat their customers, there will be no need to overwhelm people with so many choices.

This leads me to the concluding and most important statement of this book—life on demand is the way of the future and it is going to change completely what the Industrial Revolution has done for us.

We are moving from the Industrial Age, in which we learned and perfected mass production, to a more efficient age in which the accessibility to information allows us to personalize every experience and live on demand. As such, we will waste fewer resources and produce more meaningful objects.

Life on Demand and the End of Fashion Brands as We Know Them.

After reading this title, people might wonder why they had to read the entire book and get all the advice on how to survive the change, if at the end I'm going to say that this industry as we know it is going to die.

Just like with fatal patients, doctors are obligated to give them medicine. This book is my medicine, and hopefully it will make people flex their minds and think ahead. I would also prefer not to call what's coming *death*, but rather *an evolution*. However, I can hardly see how any of the elements of our business will stay the same.

What we are going through is a fundamental change of our lifestyle in which we stop consuming mass-produced products and start living life on demand, creating and consuming personalized products just when we need them. This relates to everything—food, gadgets, fashion.

In the age in which furniture is already available for 3-D printing on demand, and 3-D printers themselves become a commodity, it is only a matter of time before machines will be able to create wearable garments based on our needs and taste.

In fact, the first 3-D shoe has already been printed. In this scenario, when consumers are able to easily create their own products, the idea of a fashion brand as we know it will be completely irrelevant.

The only important thing would be the tool and materials we are using and the quality of the product.

Yes, we will still need templates and product models to inspire us and provide direction; however, the future consumers could be completely in charge of the production process, product customization and perhaps even designs.

Perhaps the store of the future will look just like a giant screen in which consumers will have a choice to customize their materials, shape and size—and get it made just a few moments later by a small 3-D printer?

As much as the thought of it sounds futuristic, it is already possible with existing technologies.

The question is, how fast will this turn into reality for the masses? This all depends on how welcoming this industry will be to change and how many developers and innovators will be willing to put their efforts into integrating their ideas into the fashion industry.

It all depends on how many designers can recognize the change, lift themselves up and stop contributing to the eighty billion garments produced around the world today in an effort to turn these garments into innovative, smart objects.

Perhaps this book can inspire a few. The market is ready for a revolution and there is no better time to start it than now.

Acknowledgements.

This book wouldn't be possible without the support of my Fashion 2.0 community of innovators. I couldn't imagine that the monthly meetup events I started back in 2008 would provide such a great source of inspiration. Now, at more than 2,400 members, this group attracts entrepreneurs and supporters who truly revolutionize the fashion industry.

Through these past few years I've seen amazing startups trying to break through the walls—founders persisting in their ideas, even when the market wasn't ready for them yet. Some of these people shared their stories with me, some reached out for advice and help, and some turned into friends.

I feel lucky to find myself in the epicenter of the fashion revolution—New York City—at this time. I'm looking forward to the next decade and hope to continue build innovative products, surrounded and inspired by the season of change.

I would also like to thank my now-husband Yanni for encouraging me to pursue my dreams, even though it means me spending gorgeous summer nights writing in a café instead of spending time together.

Lastly, I couldn't have experienced all of it without my parents, who were brave enough to face such a big change as leaving our home country, in order to build a better future for me.

CPSIA information can be obtained
at www.ICGtesting.com
Printed in the USA
LVHW021632191218
601075LV00030B/2307/P